Home Remedies

Grandma's Guide

Introduction

For this guide, I drew inspiration from the wise advice of my dear grandmother. In her times, resources were scarce, and traditional medicine was the norm. If anyone remembers any remedies or advice that Grandma used to give, like "Sorrows are less with bread" or "A good cup of tea cures everything," you're in for a treat.

1 Remedies for: Aches and Pains

In the days of yore, Grandma had a remedy for every ache and pain. From joint pains to muscle soreness, her natural remedies worked wonders.

2 Remedies for: Wounds and Cuts

Grandma's wisdom wasn't just limited to words; she knew how to heal wounds and cuts with simple, effective remedies. Her methods were tried and tested, and they always worked like magic.

3 Remedies for: Fever

Fever was no match for Grandma's knowledge. Her remedies for bringing down a fever were gentle, safe, and remarkably effective.

4 Remedies for: Flu

Facing the flu? Grandma had a solution for that too. Her flu remedies were designed to ease symptoms and help you recover faster.

5 Remedies for: Stomach Trouble

Upset stomachs were common, but Grandma had an arsenal of remedies to tackle them. From indigestion to nausea, her remedies settled the stomach in no time.

6 Remedies for: Headaches

Headaches were no joke, but Grandma knew how to make them disappear. Her remedies were soothing and provided relief, making those headaches vanish like they were never there.

Remember, these remedies might be from the past, but their effectiveness is timeless. So, the next time you're feeling under the weather, why not try one of Grandma's remedies? After all, Grandma knew best!

Remedies for Pain

1. Castor Oil: Castor oil has long been used to alleviate joint pains. Its anti-inflammatory properties are believed to reduce inflammation and pain in affected areas. You can warm some castor oil and gently massage the painful area for relief.

2. Epsom Salt Compress: Epsom salt, rich in magnesium, can be beneficial for relaxing muscles and relieving muscle pains. Add Epsom salt to a warm bath and soak in it to relax and relieve muscle tension.

3. Turmeric Tea: Turmeric contains curcumin, a compound with anti-inflammatory and analgesic properties. Making turmeric tea can help alleviate chronic pain and discomfort caused by inflammation. Mix a teaspoon of turmeric powder with hot water and honey to taste.

4. Apple Cider Vinegar Hot Compress: Apple cider vinegar can be useful for relieving muscle and joint pains. Heat some apple cider vinegar and soak a clean cloth. Then, apply it to the painful area as a hot compress.

5. Boiled Potato Compress: Potatoes contain starch, which can help reduce inflammation and pain. Boil some potatoes, mash them, and place them in a clean cloth. Apply this compress to the painful area for relief.

6. Apple Cider Vinegar and Honey: The combination of apple cider vinegar and honey can be effective in soothing sore throats. Mix a tablespoon of apple cider vinegar and a tablespoon of honey in a cup of warm water. Gargle with this mixture to alleviate irritation.

7. Eucalyptus Oil: Eucalyptus essential oil has decongestant properties and can be helpful in relieving respiratory pains. Add a few drops of eucalyptus oil to a bowl of hot water and inhale the steam to clear respiratory passages.

8. Fennel Infusion: Fennel is known for its antispasmodic properties and can relieve stomach pains as well as reduce gas formation. Prepare a fennel infusion by adding fennel seeds to hot water and let it steep before drinking.

9. Mustard Poultice: A mustard poultice can help relieve chest congestion. Mix mustard powder with flour and water to make a paste. Spread the paste on a clean cloth and apply it to the chest. Leave it on for a few minutes and then remove.

10. Olive Oil and Garlic Compress: Warm olive oil with garlic can help relieve earaches. Heat some olive oil and add a crushed garlic clove. Let the mixture cool slightly and then carefully apply it to the affected ear.

Remedies for Wounds

1. Cold Milk: Soaking a minor wound in cold milk can help alleviate pain and reduce inflammation. The cold temperature can also help soothe the affected area.

2. Cabbage Leaf Compress: Cabbage leaves can be beneficial in reducing inflammation in bruises and hematomas. Gently crush the leaves to break the fibers and then apply them to the affected area, ensuring they are in contact with the skin.

3. Calendula and Lavender Infusion: Calendula and lavender have anti-inflammatory and healing properties. Prepare an infusion with these herbs and use it to clean and disinfect minor wounds.

4. St. John's Wort Oil: St. John's Wort oil has been traditionally used to relieve minor burns and promote healing. Gently apply the oil to the wound to reap its benefits.

5. Honey with Cinnamon: Mixing honey with cinnamon can help prevent infections in cuts and scrapes. Honey has antibacterial properties, and cinnamon can enhance its effects.

6. Rosemary Essential Oil: Rosemary essential oil can be helpful in relieving headaches when massaged onto the temples and forehead. Its aromatic properties can also help relax the mind.

7. Thyme Infusion: Thyme has antibacterial properties and can help clean and disinfect wounds and cuts. Prepare a thyme infusion and use a clean cloth to apply it to the wound.

8. Cold Milk Compress: Soaking a compress in cold milk can provide relief for sunburns and soothe irritated skin.

9. Warm Saline Water: Rinsing mouth wounds with warm saline water can speed up healing and prevent infections in the mouth.

10. Lavender Oil and Honey Compress: Mix lavender oil with honey to create a soothing and antiseptic solution that you can apply to minor burns to expedite recovery.

Remedies for Fever

1. Cold Water Compresses: Cold water compresses are a quick and effective way to reduce fever. By applying them to areas such as the forehead, neck, and wrists, they help dissipate body heat and provide temporary relief. To make a compress, soak a clean cloth in cold water, gently wring it out, and place it on the mentioned areas. Change the compress when it starts to warm up.

2. Warm Water Bath: A warm water bath can be relaxing and beneficial for reducing fever. Warm water helps lower body temperature gradually without causing a sudden change that might induce chills. Avoid using water that is too cold or too hot, and make sure to dry yourself thoroughly after the bath to prevent chilling.

3. Linden Tea: Linden tea is known for its relaxing and soothing properties. It can help reduce fever and alleviate associated symptoms such as general discomfort and irritability. Prepare a cup of linden tea using dried linden flowers and drink it warm.

4. Apple Cider Vinegar Compresses: Apple cider vinegar has been traditionally used to reduce fever. Mix equal parts of apple cider vinegar and cold water and soak a clean

cloth in the solution. Then, place the compresses on the forehead, neck, and wrists to help lower body temperature.

5. Hydration: Staying well-hydrated is essential when you have a fever. The body can lose fluids due to sweating and elevated temperature. Drinking water, natural juices, and vegetable broth can prevent dehydration and aid the immune system in fighting the infection causing the fever.

6. Ginger Infusion: Ginger is known for its anti-inflammatory properties and its ability to promote blood circulation. Prepare a ginger infusion by grating a piece of fresh ginger and boiling it in water for a few minutes. Then, strain and drink the warm infusion. Besides reducing fever, ginger can relieve congestion and discomfort.

7. Light Clothing: Wearing light and breathable clothing is important when you have a fever. Light clothing allows body heat to dissipate more easily and prevents the body from overheating. Opt for natural fabrics like cotton to maintain comfort.

8. Lemon and Honey: The combination of lemon and honey in warm water is a popular home remedy to alleviate fever symptoms. Lemon provides vitamin C, which can be helpful in strengthening the immune system, while honey may have antibacterial properties and throat-soothing effects. Additionally, hydration is crucial in recovery.

9. Raw Potato Compresses: Raw potatoes have cooling properties and can help absorb body heat. Slice thin pieces of raw potato and place them on the forehead. The fresh slices will provide a sense of relief and may help reduce fever temporarily.

10. Rest: Proper rest is crucial when dealing with a fever. Allowing the body to rest and recuperate is essential for the immune system to function effectively. Avoid strenuous activities and prioritize sleep to speed up recovery.

Home Remedies for the Flu

1. Rest: When you're sick, your body needs time to recover. Proper rest allows your immune system to work more efficiently to combat the infection.

2. Hydration: Staying hydrated is crucial to loosen mucus and prevent dehydration that can occur due to fever and excessive sweating. Opt for water, homemade broths, herbal teas, and natural juices without added sugar.

3. Ginger Tea: Ginger is known for its ability to relieve congestion and reduce inflammation in the respiratory tract. You can prepare tea with fresh or powdered ginger. Besides alleviating flu symptoms, ginger tea can also warm the body and provide a comforting sensation.

4. Honey and Lemon: Honey has antibacterial properties and can help soothe the irritated throat and cough. Lemon provides vitamin C, which is beneficial for the immune system. Mixing a tablespoon of honey and the juice of half a lemon in hot water creates a soothing drink.

5. Salt Water Gargles: Warm salt water gargles can help reduce sore throat and inflammation. The saline solution can help eliminate bacteria and reduce irritation.

6. Steam: Steam inhalation can relieve nasal congestion and headaches. You can inhale steam by taking a hot shower or leaning over a bowl of hot water and covering your head with a towel to trap the steam.

7. Turmeric: Turmeric contains curcumin, a compound with anti-inflammatory and antioxidant properties. Adding a pinch of turmeric powder to warm milk can not only help alleviate flu symptoms but also provide comfort and well-being.

8. Garlic: Garlic contains allicin, a compound with antimicrobial properties. Eating raw garlic or adding it to your meals can help strengthen your immune system and fight infection.

9. Rest and Good Nutrition: Consuming nutrient-rich foods such as fruits, vegetables, lean proteins, and whole grains can provide your body with the necessary vitamins and minerals to fight infection and speed up recovery. Avoiding processed foods and high sugar content is important to maintain a healthy immune system.

10. *Avoid Tobacco and Alcohol:* Tobacco can further irritate the respiratory tract and weaken the immune system, while alcohol can dehydrate the body and affect the quality of sleep, which is essential for recovery.

Vick Vaporub

11. Vick Vaporub: Applying Vick Vaporub to the soles of the feet and rubbing it in intensely but gently, then wearing socks, can relieve cough and cold symptoms. Do this at night; it's also believed to prevent the flu.

Grandfather's Anecdote: As he used to say, there's nothing better for the flu than a good ice cream and mistreating it.

Remedies for Stomach Issues

1. Ginger Tea: Ginger contains compounds that can help reduce inflammation and alleviate stomach discomfort. You can cut or grate a small piece of fresh ginger root and boil it in water to make tea. Add a bit of honey if you desire to sweeten it.

2. Chamomile Infusion: Chamomile is known for its relaxing and anti-inflammatory properties. Prepare the infusion by steeping a chamomile tea bag in hot water for a few minutes. Drinking it after meals can help reduce indigestion.

3. Rice Water: Rice water contains starch that can help soothe the stomach lining and reduce irritation. Cook a portion of rice in water and then strain the resulting water. Drink the warm rice water.

4. Banana: Bananas are a gentle source of fiber and nutrients that can be easily tolerated by the stomach. Moreover, they contain pectin, which can help alleviate diarrhea.

5. Apple Cider Vinegar: Apple cider vinegar is acidic, but it is believed to help balance stomach pH and promote healthy digestion. Mix a tablespoon of unfiltered apple cider vinegar in a glass of water and drink it before meals.

6. Mint: Mint has soothing properties that can relieve indigestion and reduce muscle spasms in the gastrointestinal tract. You can chew fresh mint leaves, drink mint tea, or add fresh mint to your dishes.

7. Yogurt: Yogurt contains probiotics, which are beneficial bacteria for the gut. These probiotics can help improve digestive health and restore the balance of intestinal microbiota.

8. Aloe Vera: Aloe vera gel may have anti-inflammatory properties and can be helpful in soothing mild stomach irritations. Make sure to use aloe vera designed for internal consumption and follow the proper instructions for its use.

9. Cinnamon: Cinnamon can help stimulate digestion and reduce bloating by improving blood flow in the digestive system. You can add cinnamon powder to your meals or prepare cinnamon tea.

10. Warm Water with Lemon: Drinking warm water with lemon on an empty stomach can help stimulate the production of digestive enzymes and promote healthy digestion. Lemon can also help balance pH levels in the stomach.

Remedies for Headaches

1. Cold or Hot Compresses: Cold compresses can reduce inflammation by constricting blood vessels and numbing the painful area. On the other hand, hot compresses can relax tense muscles and improve blood flow. Apply a cold or hot compress on your forehead, temples, or neck for 15-20 minutes and rest. Alternate between both to see which provides more relief.

2. Massages: Massages can relax tense muscles contributing to headaches. Apply gentle pressure on your temples, forehead, and the base of your skull using circular or kneading movements. You can use your fingers or essential oils to enhance the experience.

3. Herbal Tea: Herbs like chamomile, mint, and ginger have anti-inflammatory and relaxing properties. Prepare a cup of herbal tea using dried leaves or tea bags and drink it slowly while you relax.

4. Hydration: Dehydration can trigger headaches. Make sure to drink enough water throughout the day to keep your body well-hydrated. Additionally, incorporate water-rich foods like fruits and vegetables into your diet.

5. Rest: If you're experiencing a headache, find a quiet, dark place to rest. Bright light and loud noises can worsen the pain. Resting in a calm environment can help alleviate discomfort.

6. Essential Oils: Some essential oils have relaxing and analgesic properties. Lavender can reduce tension, mint can provide a refreshing sensation, and eucalyptus can improve circulation. Dilute a few drops in a carrier oil and gently massage the affected areas.

7. Healthy Eating: Avoid foods that can trigger headaches, such as processed foods, those high in saturated fats, and high-sodium foods. Instead, opt for a balanced diet that includes fruits, vegetables, lean proteins, and whole grains.

8. Relaxation Techniques: Meditation, yoga, and deep breathing can help reduce stress and muscle tension, which, in turn, can alleviate headaches. Dedicate time each day to practice these techniques and observe if your symptoms improve over time.

9. Acupressure: Acupressure involves applying pressure to specific points on the body to relieve pain and promote well-being. A commonly used acupressure point for headaches is the area between the thumb and index finger. Gently press for a few minutes and release.

10. **Apple Cider Vinegar:** Some people have reported relief by taking a tablespoon of apple cider vinegar diluted in water. It is believed to help restore the body's acid-base balance and improve circulation. However, there is no solid scientific evidence supporting this claim, so it's important to keep this in mind.

Remember, if headaches are frequent, severe, or interfering with your quality of life, it's advisable to seek the advice of a healthcare professional for an accurate diagnosis and personalized treatment.

Please note that these remedies are alternative approaches and not a substitute for professional medical advice.

The Grandma's

Herbal Guide

1. Chamomile (Matricaria chamomilla)

2. Peppermint (Mentha piperita)

3. Aloe Vera

4. Echinacea (Echinacea purpurea)

5. Ginseng (Panax ginseng)

6. Turmeric (Curcuma longa)

7. Valerian (Valeriana officinalis)

8. Sage (Salvia officinalis)

9. Ginkgo Biloba

10. Rosemary (Rosmarinus officinalis)

11. Marigold (Calendula officinalis)

"The Grandma's Herbal Guide

Medicinal plants have been used for centuries in various cultures around the world to treat a wide variety of conditions and illnesses. Below, I present to you some common medicinal plants and their therapeutic functions."

Chamomile

Chamomile (*Matricaria chamomilla*) is a medicinal plant known for its calming and anti-inflammatory properties. Its main active components include:

1. Chamomile essential oil: Contains compounds like bisabolol and alpha-bisabolol oxide, which have anti-inflammatory and soothing properties.

2. Flavonoids: These compounds have antioxidant and anti-inflammatory properties that can help reduce inflammation and protect against oxidative damage.

3. Volatile oils: Include components like alpha-bisabolol, contributing to chamomile's anti-inflammatory and calming properties.

Common uses of chamomile include:

1. Digestive disorders: Chamomile is used to alleviate digestive problems such as stomach discomfort, gas, indigestion, and heartburn. It can help calm the gastrointestinal system.

2. Insomnia and anxiety: Chamomile has mild sedative properties and is used to promote sleep and relieve anxiety. It can be consumed as tea before bedtime to induce relaxation.

3. Skin conditions: Chamomile is used in creams and lotions to treat mild burns, irritations, rashes, and insect bites. Its anti-inflammatory and healing properties can soothe irritated skin.

4. Relief of eye irritation: Chamomile is sometimes used as an eye drop to relieve eye irritation and reduce inflammation.

5. Relief of menstrual symptoms: Some women find relief in consuming chamomile to reduce menstrual symptoms such as cramps and general discomfort.

It is important to note that while chamomile is generally safe for most people when consumed as tea or applied topically, some individuals may be allergic to it. Additionally, if you are pregnant or taking medications, it is advisable to consult a healthcare professional before using it for medicinal purposes.

Note:

1. Possible allergies: Like any medicinal plant or food, some people may be allergic to chamomile. If you experience symptoms such as rashes, itching, swelling, or difficulty breathing after consuming or applying chamomile, you should discontinue its use and seek medical advice.

2. Pregnancy and breastfeeding: If you are pregnant or breastfeeding, it is important to consult a healthcare professional before consuming chamomile for medicinal purposes. Although it is generally considered safe in moderate amounts, specific guidance is prudent due to possible interactions or unwanted effects.

3. Drug interactions: Chamomile may interact with certain medications, such as anticoagulants and sedatives. If you are taking medications, especially regularly, consult your doctor before starting to use chamomile as a complementary treatment.

4. Proper preparation: Ensure you prepare and consume chamomile properly. If you are using it as tea, follow the preparation instructions and do not exceed the recommended doses.

It is always wise to be aware of the possible contraindications and side effects of any medicinal herb or plant and seek medical guidance when necessary. Moreover, if you experience an adverse reaction to consuming or applying chamomile, seek medical attention immediately.

Peppermint

Peppermint (Mentha piperita) is a medicinal plant known for its refreshing, digestive, and calming properties. Its main active components include essential oils, such as menthol, which give it its therapeutic properties. Here are more details about its functions and uses:

1. Relief of Digestive Disorders:

   - Indigestion: Peppermint is commonly used to relieve indigestion as it can help relax the muscles of the gastrointestinal tract, facilitating digestion. Menthol in peppermint can also relieve the feeling of stomach heaviness.

   - Gas and Flatulence: Consuming peppermint can reduce abdominal bloating and gas. It can help calm the gastrointestinal tract and promote the release of trapped gas.

2. Soothing Properties:

   - Menthol in peppermint has calming and refreshing properties. It can help relieve throat irritation and provide a fresh sensation when consumed as tea or inhaled through peppermint essential oil vapors.

3. Headache Relief:

- Application of diluted peppermint essential oil on the temples or forehead can help relieve tension headaches and migraines due to its relaxing and vasodilating properties.

4. Treatment of Cold Symptoms and Nasal Congestion:

  - Peppermint can relieve nasal congestion and reduce throat irritation when its vapor is inhaled or consumed as tea. It is also found in many congestion relief products.

5. Culinary Use:

  - Peppermint is used in cooking to add flavor and aroma to a variety of dishes and beverages, such as salads, mint tea, cocktails, and desserts.

It is important to note that although peppermint is generally safe when consumed in moderate amounts, high concentrations of menthol can cause irritation in some individuals. If you have chronic gastrointestinal issues or allergies, it's advisable to consult a healthcare professional before using peppermint for medicinal purposes. Additionally, ensure you properly dilute peppermint essential oils if you plan to apply them to the skin.

Note:

1. Moderate Consumption and Precautions: While peppermint is generally safe in moderate amounts, high concentrations of menthol can cause irritation, especially in individuals with chronic gastrointestinal issues or allergies. It's advisable to consult a healthcare professional before using peppermint for medicinal purposes, especially if you have preexisting health concerns.

2. Peppermint Essential Oils: When applying peppermint essential oils to the skin, it's important to dilute them properly with a carrier oil, such as sweet almond oil, to avoid irritations or allergic reactions. The skin can be sensitive, and applying undiluted essential oils can be too strong.

Peppermint is a versatile and widely used herb, but as with any medicinal plant or herb, it's important to use it responsibly and be aware of possible side effects or contraindications. Seeking medical guidance is always advisable when you have specific concerns about its use, especially for topical applications or significant consumption.

Aloe Vera

Aloe vera is a plant that has been used for centuries worldwide for its medicinal properties. Its most common uses and therapeutic functions include:

1. Healing and Anti-inflammatory Properties:

- Aloe vera gel, extracted from the plant's leaves, is known for its healing and anti-inflammatory properties. It is used to accelerate the healing of minor wounds, mild burns, cuts, and abrasions. Applying the gel to the affected skin can help reduce inflammation and promote tissue regeneration.

2. Skin Irritations:

- Aloe vera is used to soothe skin irritations such as sunburns, rashes, insect bites, and mild dermatitis. Its calming and refreshing properties can provide relief to irritated skin.

3. Digestive Issues:

- Consuming aloe vera juice, obtained from the inner part of the leaves, has been traditionally used to treat digestive problems like constipation and gastrointestinal irritation. It has mild laxative properties that can help relieve occasional constipation.

4. Skin Hydration:

   - Aloe vera gel is an excellent skin moisturizer. It is used in skincare products like creams and lotions to keep the skin soft and hydrated.

5. Chronic Skin Conditions:

   - Some people use aloe vera to treat chronic skin conditions such as eczema and psoriasis. Although it doesn't cure these conditions, it can provide temporary relief from itching and irritation.

6. Hair Care:

   - Aloe vera is also used in hair care products like shampoos and conditioners due to its ability to hydrate and strengthen hair.

It's important to note that while aloe vera is generally safe for topical use and in moderate amounts for digestive issues, its consumption in large quantities or over a prolonged period is not recommended as it can cause side effects such as diarrhea and electrolyte imbalances. If you have a medical condition or are taking medications, it's advisable to consult a healthcare professional before using aloe vera for medicinal purposes.

Additionally, make sure to perform a patch test on a small area before applying aloe vera to a larger skin surface to ensure there are no allergic reactions.

Note:

1. Moderate Consumption and Precautions: If using aloe vera for digestive problems, it's important to consume it in moderate amounts and follow dosage recommendations. Excessive consumption of aloe vera can lead to side effects like diarrhea and electrolyte imbalances.

2. Consult a Healthcare Professional: If you have an existing medical condition, are taking medications, or are pregnant, it's essential to consult a healthcare professional before using aloe vera for medicinal purposes. There might be medication interactions or specific contraindications to consider.

3. Patch Test: Before applying aloe vera to a large skin area, especially for people with sensitive skin, it's a good practice to perform a patch test in a small area to ensure there are no allergic reactions or irritation. This is especially important when using aloe vera directly from the plant.

Aloe vera can be beneficial for many people in treating skin conditions and mild digestive problems, but like any natural remedy, it's important to use it with caution and responsibility. Always be aware of possible contraindications and side effects and seek professional guidance when needed.

Echinacea

Echinacea (Echinacea purpurea) is a widely known medicinal plant renowned for its immune system-boosting properties. Its primary function is to strengthen the immune system and is used for preventing and treating colds and other infections. Here is more information about its uses and benefits:

1. Immune System Stimulation:

- Echinacea contains bioactive compounds such as polysaccharides and alkamides that can stimulate the immune system. It is believed that this plant increases the production of white blood cells, such as macrophages and lymphocytes, which are essential for fighting infections.

2. Prevention and Treatment of Colds and Similar Illnesses:

- Echinacea is commonly used to prevent colds and reduce the duration and severity of symptoms when a cold has already developed. It can shorten the cold period and alleviate symptoms such as nasal congestion, sore throat, and fever.

3. Support in Respiratory Infections:

- Besides colds, Echinacea is often used in the treatment of respiratory infections such as bronchitis and sinusitis.

4. Urinary Tract Infections:

  - Some people use Echinacea for treating urinary tract infections, although its effectiveness in this regard is less clear compared to its use for respiratory infections.

5. Minor Wounds and Burns:

  - Topically applied, Echinacea extract can help accelerate the healing of minor wounds and burns due to its anti-inflammatory and antimicrobial properties.

It's important to note that scientific studies on the efficacy of Echinacea have yielded mixed results, and its use is not without controversy. Some research suggests it might be useful in preventing and treating colds, while others have not found significant benefits. Additionally, the quality and preparation of Echinacea products can vary, affecting their efficacy.

If you're considering using Echinacea to treat or prevent an illness, it's advisable to consult a healthcare professional, especially if you have allergies or are taking other medications, as there could be potential interactions. Furthermore, Echinacea should not be used as a substitute for proper medical treatment in severe cases of infection or illness.

Scientific Studies on the Efficacy of Echinacea:

Research on medicinal plants, including Echinacea, can be complex due to various factors such as differences in Echinacea species used, parts of the plant utilized, dosages, preparation methods, and study populations. Here are some additional considerations:

Note:

1. Variety of Species and Plant Parts: There are several Echinacea species, such as Echinacea purpurea, Echinacea angustifolia, and Echinacea pallida, and their chemical profiles and properties can vary. Additionally, different parts of the plant, such as roots, leaves, and flowers, may contain different active compounds.

2. Dosage and Treatment Duration: Dosage and treatment duration can influence results. Some studies might use higher or lower doses, which could affect outcomes. Also, the

timing of Echinacea intake (e.g., at the onset of a cold versus over an extended period) can influence its perceived effectiveness.

3. Interactions with Other Medications and Medical Conditions: Interactions with other medications and participants' underlying medical conditions can influence outcomes. It's important to consider Echinacea's safety and suitability for each individual.

4. Quality and Preparation of the Product: The quality of Echinacea products can vary by manufacturer and preparation method. Product quality and potency can affect effectiveness.

5. Individual Response: Response to Echinacea and other herbs can vary from person to person. Some individuals may experience significant benefits, while others may not notice any improvement.

In summary, if you decide to use Echinacea for medicinal purposes, it's important to do so knowledgeably. Consult a healthcare professional for specific guidance and ensure it is safe and suitable for your individual needs. Additionally, seek out quality products and follow the manufacturer's dosage recommendations. As with any supplement or herb, it is crucial to be critical and aware of available research and maintain realistic expectations about its potential benefits.

Ginseng

Ginseng, specifically Panax ginseng, is a widely recognized medicinal plant in traditional Asian medicine, especially in Chinese and Korean medicine. It has several potential health benefits, and its prominent functions include:

1. Increased Energy and Stamina:

- Ginseng has traditionally been used as a natural tonic to boost energy and stamina. It can help combat fatigue and enhance both physical and mental endurance, making it a popular choice for those seeking an energy boost.

2. Improved Cognitive Function:

- Ginseng has also been associated with improvements in cognitive function, such as memory, concentration, and mental performance. It is believed to stimulate the central nervous system and have positive effects on brain activity.

3. Adaptogenic Properties:

- Ginseng is often classified as an adaptogen, meaning it can help the body adapt to stress and restore balance. It is believed to act on the endocrine system and the immune system to enhance the body's stress response and promote homeostasis.

4. *Enhanced Sexual Function:*

   - Ginseng has also been traditionally used as an aphrodisiac and to improve sexual function in both men and women. Some studies suggest it may have benefits for erectile dysfunction and libido.

It's important to highlight that there are different types of ginseng, such as Panax ginseng (Asian ginseng), Panax quinquefolius (American ginseng), and others. Each type may have different properties and concentrations of active compounds, so it's important to choose the right type based on your needs and health goals.

Additionally, the use of ginseng should be supervised with caution as it can have side effects and may interact with certain medications. If you're considering using ginseng for medicinal purposes, it's advisable to consult a healthcare professional for specific guidance to ensure it's safe and suitable for you.

You're absolutely right; it's crucial to consider that there are different types of ginseng, each with slightly different properties and benefits due to their unique chemical compositions. Here's a brief description of some of the most common types of ginseng:

Note:

1. Panax ginseng (Asian Ginseng):

   - One of the most well-known and widely used types of ginseng.

   - Believed to have stimulating properties that can increase energy and stamina.

   - Traditionally used to improve concentration and cognitive function.

   - Also considered an adaptogen, aiding in stress reduction and improving stress resistance.

2. Panax quinquefolius (American Ginseng):

   - Often used as an alternative to Asian ginseng, although its properties might be less potent.

   - Associated with improvements in immune function and stress resistance.

   - Like Asian ginseng, it's considered an adaptogen and is used to combat fatigue and exhaustion.

3. Eleutherococcus senticosus (Siberian Ginseng):

   - Despite its common name, it's not a true ginseng but is called so due to its similar adaptogenic properties.

   - Used to increase both physical and mental endurance, enhance concentration and mental clarity, and alleviate stress.

- Some people prefer it due to its safety profile and lower cost compared to Asian ginseng.

4. Other Types of Ginseng:

- In addition to the ones mentioned above, there are other lesser-known types of ginseng, such as Japanese ginseng (Panax japonicus) and Indian ginseng (Withania somnifera, also known as Ashwagandha).

- Each of these ginsengs can have unique properties and is traditionally used in different cultures for a variety of purposes.

When choosing a type of ginseng, it's important to research and consider your specific health needs and goals, as well as consult with a healthcare professional or herbalist for proper guidance. Additionally, be aware that the quality and concentration of ginseng products can vary, so it's important to choose high-quality products from reputable sources if you decide to use ginseng for medicinal purposes.

Turmeric

Turmeric (Curcuma longa) is a spice and medicinal plant that has been used for centuries in traditional medicine, especially in Ayurvedic and Hindu medicine, due to its therapeutic properties. Its key functions and benefits include:

1. Anti-inflammatory Properties: Turmeric contains an active compound called curcumin, which has been shown to have potent anti-inflammatory properties. It is used to alleviate inflammation and has been researched in the context of chronic inflammatory conditions such as rheumatoid arthritis.

2. Antioxidant Properties: Curcumin also acts as an antioxidant, meaning it can help combat oxidative stress in the body by neutralizing free radicals. This can have overall health benefits and help prevent premature aging and some chronic diseases.

3. Pain Relief: Turmeric has traditionally been used to relieve pain, especially in musculoskeletal conditions. Some people find pain relief in cases of arthritis, headaches, and other types of chronic pain by consuming turmeric.

4. Brain Health: Curcumin has been suggested to have benefits for brain health, including improving cognitive function and protecting against neurodegenerative diseases such as Alzheimer's. However, more research is needed in this area.

5. Heart Health: The role of turmeric in cardiovascular health has been studied, and some research suggests it could help reduce the risk of heart diseases by improving endothelial function and reducing inflammation.

It's important to note that turmeric is generally safe when consumed in moderate amounts as part of the diet. However, curcumin has limited bioavailability, meaning it can be challenging for the body to absorb and utilize efficiently when consumed alone. Therefore, it is often recommended to consume turmeric in combination with black pepper, which contains piperine, a compound that can enhance the absorption of curcumin.

Note:

1. Limited Bioavailability of Curcumin: Curcumin, the active compound in turmeric with beneficial properties, has limited bioavailability, meaning the body struggles to efficiently absorb and utilize it when consumed alone.

2. Piperine in Black Pepper: Piperine is a compound found in black pepper and has been shown to significantly enhance the absorption of curcumin in the body. Piperine helps prevent curcumin from breaking down rapidly in the digestive tract, allowing better absorption into the bloodstream.

3. Combination of Turmeric and Black Pepper: To maximize the benefits of turmeric, many people consume turmeric in combination with black pepper. This can be achieved by adding freshly ground black pepper to foods containing turmeric or by taking supplements that combine turmeric and piperine.

4. Turmeric Supplements with Piperine: Turmeric supplements that include piperine to enhance curcumin absorption are also available in the market. These supplements are often marketed as "optimized curcumin" or "turmeric with piperine."

It's important to highlight that if you're considering taking turmeric supplements for therapeutic purposes, it's advisable to consult a healthcare professional, especially if you're taking medications, as curcumin could interact with some of them. Additionally, maintaining balance and not exceeding recommended doses is important to avoid unwanted side effects. The combination of turmeric and black pepper is an effective strategy to enhance curcumin absorption and make the most of its health benefits.

Valerian

Valerian (Valeriana officinalis) is a medicinal plant that has been used for centuries as a natural sedative and relaxant. Its primary functions and uses include:

1. Natural Sedative:

   - Valerian is known for its ability to act as a natural sedative. It is used to relieve insomnia and improve sleep quality. It can help reduce sleep latency (the time it takes to fall asleep) and decrease the number of nighttime awakenings.

2. Treatment of Anxiety and Stress:

   - Valerian is used to treat anxiety and stress due to its calming effects. It can help reduce anxiety symptoms such as restlessness and muscle tension.

3. Muscle Relaxation:

   - In addition to its sedative properties, valerian is also used to relax muscles and relieve muscle tension. This can be helpful for people experiencing muscle spasms or contractions due to stress.

4. Relief of Menopausal Symptoms:

- Some women use valerian to alleviate menopausal symptoms such as hot flashes and irritability, due to its ability to reduce anxiety and promote relaxation.

5. Restless Legs Syndrome (RLS):

   - Valerian has also been used in the treatment of Restless Legs Syndrome (RLS), a condition characterized by the need to move the legs due to uncomfortable sensations. It can help alleviate symptoms and improve sleep quality in people with RLS.

Valerian is available in various forms, including capsules, tablets, tinctures, and tea. It is important to note that while valerian is generally considered safe, it can have sedative effects, so it's important not to drive or engage in activities that require concentration after consumption. Additionally, it is recommended to use it under the supervision of a healthcare professional, especially if you are taking other medications or have preexisting medical conditions. The appropriate dosage and duration of treatment should be determined by a healthcare professional.

Note:

1. *Forms of Presentation:* Valerian is available in various forms, allowing people to choose the one that best suits their preferences and needs. Capsules, tablets, tinctures, and valerian tea are some common options.

2. *Sedative Effects:* Valerian is known for its sedative and relaxing effects. It can help induce sleep and alleviate anxiety, but this also means it can cause drowsiness. Therefore, it is important to avoid activities that require concentration, such as driving or operating machinery, after consuming valerian.

3. *Supervision of a Healthcare Professional:* If you are considering using valerian for medicinal purposes, especially regularly or in high doses, it is advisable to consult a healthcare professional. This is especially important if you are taking other medications or have preexisting medical conditions, as there might be interactions or contraindications.

4. *Appropriate Dosage and Duration of Treatment:* The appropriate dosage of valerian can vary from person to person and depending on the purpose of use. A healthcare professional can provide guidance on the proper dosage and duration of treatment. It is important to follow these recommendations to avoid unwanted side effects or dependence.

5. Responsible Use: As with any herb or supplement, it is fundamental to use valerian responsibly and consciously. Do not exceed recommended doses and do not use it as a substitute for proper medical treatment in the case of serious medical conditions.

Valerian can be a useful option for people seeking relief from anxiety, insomnia, and stress, but it is important to use it cautiously and under appropriate guidance to ensure its safe and effective use. Like with any supplement or herb, the safety and suitability of valerian use can vary from person to person, making the supervision of a healthcare professional a prudent measure.

Sage

Sage (Salvia officinalis) is a medicinal herb that has been used for a long time due to its various properties and health benefits. Its primary functions and uses include:

1. Antimicrobial Properties:

- Sage contains antimicrobial compounds such as essential oils and flavonoids, which can help fight bacterial and fungal infections. It has been traditionally used to treat digestive problems caused by infections and for mouth rinses to address oral health issues.

2. Antioxidant Properties:

- Sage is rich in antioxidants, which help combat oxidative stress in the body and can protect cells and tissues from damage caused by free radicals. This can contribute to overall health and healthy aging.

3. Digestive Problems:

- Sage has been used to treat a variety of digestive issues such as indigestion, flatulence, colic, and diarrhea. Its antimicrobial properties can help alleviate gastrointestinal infections.

4. Sore Throats and Oral Conditions:

  - Sage has been used in mouth rinses and gargles to relieve sore throat, gum inflammation, and other oral conditions. Its antimicrobial and anti-inflammatory properties can be beneficial in this regard.

5. Menopausal Symptoms:

  - Some women use sage to alleviate menopausal symptoms such as hot flashes and night sweats. Phytoestrogens present in sage are believed to help balance hormones during this period.

6. Memory and Concentration Enhancement:

  - Some studies have investigated the possibility that sage can enhance memory and concentration, although more research is needed to confirm these effects.

Sage can be used in various forms, including as tea infusion, in capsules, tinctures, or essential oils. As with any herb or supplement, it's important to use it responsibly and under proper supervision. If you have preexisting medical conditions or are taking other medications, it's advisable to consult a healthcare professional before using sage for medicinal purposes. The appropriate dosage and duration of treatment should be determined by a healthcare professional.

Note:

1. *Forms of Presentation: Sage can be used in various forms, including tea infusion, capsules, tinctures, or essential oils. The choice of presentation form will depend on personal preferences and treatment goals.*

2. *Responsibility in Use: It is fundamental to use sage and other supplements or herbs responsibly. This includes respecting recommended doses and following the product instructions or recommendations from a healthcare professional.*

3. *Consultation with a Healthcare Professional: If you have preexisting medical conditions, are taking other medications, or have concerns about using sage for medicinal purposes, it's advisable to consult a healthcare professional. They can provide personalized guidance and ensure that sage is safe and suitable for your individual needs.*

4. *Dosage and Duration of Treatment: The appropriate dosage and duration of treatment can vary based on the purpose of use and the individual. A healthcare professional can help determine the correct dosage and optimal usage period.*

5. Potency and Quality of the Product: When selecting sage products, make sure to choose high-quality options from reputable sources. Potency and quality can vary between products, so it's important to obtain products from trusted sources.

6. Side Effects and Contraindications: While sage is generally safe when used correctly, some individuals might experience side effects, or there might be contraindications in specific cases. A healthcare professional can help identify and manage these potential issues.

The use of medicinal herbs such as sage can be beneficial for many people, but it is crucial to do so in an informed manner and under supervision when necessary. Guidance from a healthcare professional can provide peace of mind and ensure the safe and effective use of sage or other natural remedies.

Ginkgo Biloba

Ginkgo biloba is a herb known for its properties that improve blood circulation and its use in the treatment of cognitive disorders. Here is an expanded explanation of its function and use:

1. Improved Blood Circulation: Ginkgo biloba has been traditionally used to enhance blood circulation, especially in the brain and extremities. This is due to its ability to dilate blood vessels and improve blood flow. Improved blood circulation can have several health benefits.

2. Enhanced Cognitive Function: Ginkgo biloba has been studied in relation to improving cognitive function, especially in older individuals. By increasing blood flow to the brain and acting as an antioxidant, it is believed to help preserve brain function, enhance memory, and mental clarity.

3. Treatment of Dementia and Memory Disorders: Ginkgo biloba has been used in the treatment of dementia, including Alzheimer's disease, and in memory disorders such as

mild cognitive impairment related to aging. However, its effectiveness in these cases can vary and is the subject of ongoing research.

It is important to note that while Ginkgo biloba is used to treat cognitive problems, it is not a definitive cure for dementia or Alzheimer's disease. Additionally, its use should be supervised by a healthcare professional, as it can interact with other medications and may have side effects in some individuals.

The appropriate dosage and duration of treatment should be determined in consultation with a healthcare professional. As with any supplement or herb, safety and efficacy are important, and it is essential to use Ginkgo biloba responsibly and under proper supervision.

Note:

1. **Not a Definitive Cure:** Ginkgo biloba is used to enhance cognitive function and treat memory disorders, but it is not a definitive cure for dementia or Alzheimer's disease. Its effects can vary from person to person, and its ability to delay the progression of these conditions is not guaranteed.

2. **Professional Supervision:** The use of Ginkgo biloba should be supervised by a healthcare professional, especially if you are taking other medications. It can interact with certain medications, such as anticoagulants, and increase the risk of bleeding. Additionally, some individuals may experience side effects, such as headaches, gastrointestinal disturbances, or allergies, making medical supervision essential.

3. **Product Safety and Quality:** Ensure you obtain high-quality Ginkgo biloba products from reliable sources. Quality and potency can vary between products and manufacturers, so it's important to choose products that are safe and effective.

4. Proper Dosage: The appropriate dosage of Ginkgo biloba can vary based on the individual and the condition being treated. A healthcare professional can provide guidance on the correct dosage and duration of treatment.

5. Side Effects and Contraindications: Some individuals may experience side effects or be allergic to Ginkgo biloba. Additionally, it should be avoided before surgery due to its potential anticoagulant effect. A healthcare professional can help identify and manage these potential issues.

In summary, Ginkgo biloba can be an option for enhancing cognitive function in certain individuals, but it must be used responsibly, supervised, and with awareness of its possible limitations. Consulting with a healthcare professional is a prudent step before using it, especially if a serious medical condition is being treated. Safety and suitability of Ginkgo biloba use can vary from person to person, so taking appropriate precautions is essential.

Rosemary

Rosemary (Rosmarinus officinalis) is a herb known for its precise uses, emphasizing its versatility in traditional medicine and herbalism. Here are the key points highlighted:

1. Antioxidant and Anti-inflammatory Properties: Rosemary is known to be a rich source of antioxidants, which can help combat oxidative stress in the body. Additionally, its anti-inflammatory properties can be beneficial in reducing inflammation in the body.

2. Memory Enhancement: Rosemary has been studied in relation to memory and concentration improvement. The aroma of rosemary has been associated in studies with increased mental alertness and cognitive function. Some people use rosemary essential oils to help improve concentration during study or work.

3. Muscle Pain Relief: Rosemary has been traditionally used to relieve muscle pain and tension. Rosemary essential oils can be diluted and applied in massages to help relax muscles and alleviate pain.

4. Improved Blood Circulation: Rosemary is believed to improve blood circulation by dilating blood vessels. This can be beneficial for cardiovascular health and help carry more oxygen and nutrients to tissues.

It's important to note that while rosemary has these potential health benefits, its effectiveness can vary from person to person and depending on the method of use. Additionally, if you are considering using rosemary essential oils on the skin, it's important to dilute them properly and consider possible skin sensitivities.

As with any supplement or herb, it's important to use rosemary responsibly and take precautions, especially if you have preexisting medical conditions or are considering its use in concentrated forms such as essential oils. Consulting with a healthcare professional if you have doubts or concerns is a prudent step to ensure safe and effective use of rosemary.

Note:

1. *Variability in Effectiveness: Like many natural herbs and supplements, the effectiveness of rosemary can vary from person to person. What works well for one person might not work the same way for another. It's important to be aware that results can be subjective and may require time to notice.*

2. *Proper Dilution of Essential Oils: If you decide to use rosemary essential oils on the skin, it is crucial to properly dilute them before application. Essential oils are highly concentrated and can cause irritation or skin sensitivity if applied directly to the skin without dilution. Using a carrier oil, such as sweet almond oil or coconut oil, to dilute rosemary essential oil before applying it to the skin is recommended.*

3. *Skin Sensitivities: Each person can have different skin sensitivities. Before applying any essential oil over a large area of the skin, it is wise to perform a patch test in a small area to ensure there are no adverse reactions, such as redness, itching, or irritation.*

4. *Consultation with a Healthcare Professional: If you have any concerns or doubts about using rosemary or rosemary essential oils, it is advisable to consult with a healthcare*

professional or an aromatherapist. They can provide specific and personalized guidance on the safe and effective use of these products.

In general, safety and effectiveness are paramount when using herbs and essential oils for medicinal or therapeutic purposes. Individuality and caution are key, and conducting preliminary tests to avoid adverse reactions is important. Seeking professional guidance when using herbs and essential oils on the skin or for health purposes is always advisable.

Calendula

Calendula (Calendula officinalis) and its uses are precise, highlighting its beneficial properties in skincare and the treatment of wounds and skin conditions. Here are the key points emphasized:

1. Anti-inflammatory and Healing Properties: Calendula is known for its anti-inflammatory properties, which can help reduce inflammation in the skin, and its healing properties, which can promote wound and burn healing. These properties make calendula useful in treating a variety of skin issues.

2. Wound and Burn Treatment: Calendula has been traditionally used to treat minor wounds, burns, and abrasions. It can help speed up the skin healing process and reduce the risk of infection.

3. Skin Rashes and Skin Issues: In addition to wounds and burns, calendula has been used to treat skin rashes, irritations, eczema, and other dermatological conditions. Its soothing properties can relieve discomfort and itching associated with these conditions.

4. Forms of Use: Calendula can be found in various forms such as ointments, salves, creams, oils, and tinctures. It can also be used to make tea infusions or compresses. The choice of the form of use depends on the condition and personal preference.

5. Patch Test: As with any new product applied to the skin, it's important to conduct a patch test on a small area before applying calendula to a larger area of the skin. This helps ensure there are no allergic reactions or irritation.

In summary, calendula is a versatile herb widely used in skincare and the treatment of minor wounds, burns, skin rashes, and other dermatological problems. Its anti-inflammatory and healing properties make it valuable in the first aid kit and general skincare. As always, it's important to use it responsibly and consult a healthcare professional if you have serious skin conditions or concerns about its use.

Note:

Calendula is widely recognized for its anti-inflammatory and healing properties, making it a valuable choice for first aid kits and overall skincare. However, it's essential to use it responsibly, following application guidelines, and if necessary, consulting with a healthcare professional, especially in cases of serious skin conditions or doubts about its use.

Note:

It's important to emphasize that if you choose to use medicinal plants to treat any condition, you should do so with caution and consult a healthcare professional or an experienced herbalist. This is because some plants can interact with medications or have side effects. Furthermore, proper dosage and preparation methods are also crucial to ensure their safety and effectiveness. Consulting with an expert is essential for the responsible and safe use of medicinal herbs.

Dedication:

To: My Grandmother Asuncion

Author:

Monica Alonso